HOLIDAY DEPRESSION

HOW TO OVERCOME HOLIDAY DEPRESSION AND ADDICTION

By Patricia A Carlisle

Introduction

I want to thank you and congratulate you for choosing the book, *"HOLIDAY DEPRESSION: How to Overcome Depression and Addiction"*.

This book contains proven steps and strategies on how to overcome depression, and the compulsion to spend during the holidays.

The holiday season often brings unwelcome guests-stress and depression. And it's no wonder. The holidays present a dizzying array of demands – parties, shopping, baking, cleaning and entertaining, to name just a few. Feeling down during the holidays can be tough, especially since you seem so out of step with the world. Everyone else seems to be beaming, rosy-cheeked, bursting with holiday spirit. You're feeling wretched and exhausted.

Holidays are supposed to be a time of joy and celebration, but for many people they are anything but. Depression may occur at any time of the year, but the stress and anxiety of the holiday season, especially during the months of November and December (and to a lesser extent, just before Valentine's Day), may cause even those who are usually content to experience loneliness and a lack of fulfillment.

According to one 2015 American study of patients treated by emergency psychiatric services during the Christmas season, the most common stressors were feelings of loneliness and being without a family.

Thanks again for choosing this book, I hope you enjoy it!

ABOUT THE AUTHOR

Patricia A. Carlisle, MSW, CBT

Patricia Carlisle- a Master in Social Work and Cognitive Behavioral Therapist (CBT) gives out an expression of how important it is for an individual to take into consideration the concept of self-assessment to know what human, technical and conceptual skills they posses to perform or to achieve what they desire, or to deal with everyday life. However, every particular group of people has their own unique set of ideas, traditions and events including the frame of mind according to which people perform but there are many who faces problems and fail to maintain a healthy mind set affecting their behaviors and performance to those around them.

> People like Patricia Carlisle are among those who have felt this urge of serving people and helping them out of their mental crisis towards a healthy life. She has experienced some close encounters in her personal life regarding mental health issues in her family and friends that has encouraged her to pursue this as her career.

Currently Patricia Carlisle is serving as a Certified On-Line Cognitive Behavioral Therapist with an extensive 15years of experience using Cognitive-Behavior Therapy Techniques. She envisions a world where everyone gets mental health treatment with no mental health stigma and to make it real she has already set up her own Holistic Measure Online Comprehensive Behavioral Healthcare Company after retiring from The Nord Center in The Partial Hospitalization Program (PHP) Dept for 5 years and Murtis H. Taylor Mental Health Center as a mental health counselor, psychological support technician and case manager for 10 years to emulsify her skills more professionally.

Along with this, she has wrote down her passion as a clinician in 25 or more short books to help individuals and families get their life back, freeing them of the restraints of negative thinking, anxiety and depression by using different approaches. She is highly appreciated among her clients for her flexibility and professionalism of dealing with them graciously. To reach her, make use of her direct website address: http://therapist2013.wix.com/e-therapy . As she is ready to inspire hope and contribute to health and well-being by providing the best online health care through comprehensive practice, education and research.

TABLE OF CONTENT

Chapter 1

THE HOLIDAY SUICIDE MYTH

The myth has been repeated so many times, most people consider it common knowledge, and more people commit suicide between Thanksgiving and Christmas than at any other time of the year. Although it sounds reasonable, it simply isn't true.

Contrary to popular belief, December actually has the fewest suicide attempts of any month of the year. The facts, while seemingly encouraging, may be more complicated. While it's true that suicide attempts tend to drop off just before and during the holidays, there is a significant rising in suicide rates following Christmas – a 40 percent rising, according to one large Danish study. Christmas it-self seems to have a protective effect with regard to certain types of psychopathology, say researchers, but there is a significant rebound effect immediately following the holiday.

Although fewer people utilize emergency services, or attempt suicide during December, there is an increase in certain other kinds of psychopathology, including mood disorders such as dysphoria (feeling of sadness), and substance abuse.

Chapter 2

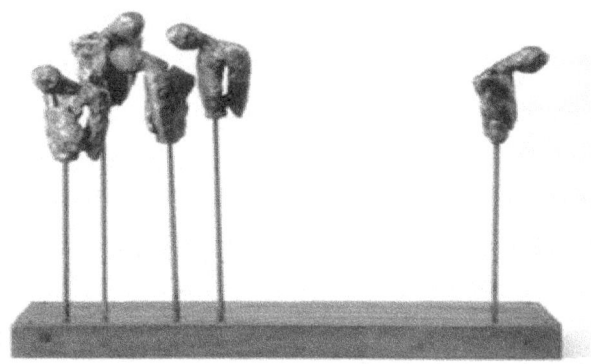

SOCIAL ISOLATION

Social isolation is one of the biggest predictors of depression especially during the holidays. People who are lonely, or have feelings of disconnectedness often avoid social interactions at holiday time. Unfortunately, withdrawing often exacerbates the feelings of loneliness and symptoms of depression. These individuals may see other people spending time with friends and family and ask themselves. "Why can't that be me?", or "Why is everyone else so much happier than I am"?

Experts advise a regimen of self-care during the holidays, which includes eating a healthy diet, maintaining a regular sleep pattern, and exercise. In fact, as little as 30-minutes of cardiovascular exercise can provide an immediate mood boost similar to the effects of an antidepressant medications.

One of the best things a person can do, however, is to reach out to others despite how difficult it may seem. That loneliness should act in a similar way to thirst, motivating you to change your behavior in some way.

Chapter 3

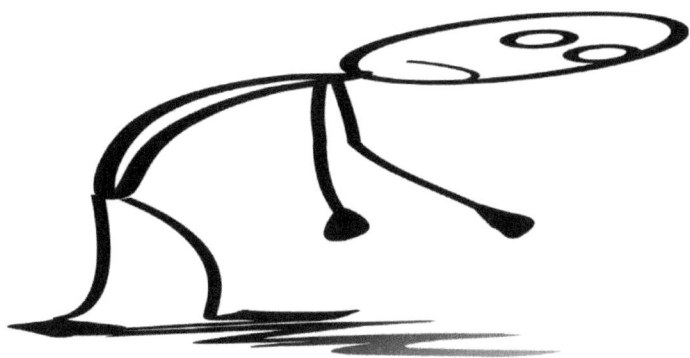

GRIEVING DURING THE HOLIDAYS

For many people, holidays are a painful reminder of what once was. This is especially true for people who have experienced a significant loss such as the death of a spouse or a break-up. For these individuals, it is important to manage expectations, experts say.

When envisioning how the holidays will unfold after a loss, a person should include both the highs and lows in his or her expectations. Valentine's Day can be especially difficult for people who've ended a relationship.

Don't let anyone put a time limit on your broken heart, comforting experiences such as going for a walk, eating well, and keeping a routine sleep schedule. Experts stresses that people going through this type of grieving shouldn't feel ashamed.

Chapter 4

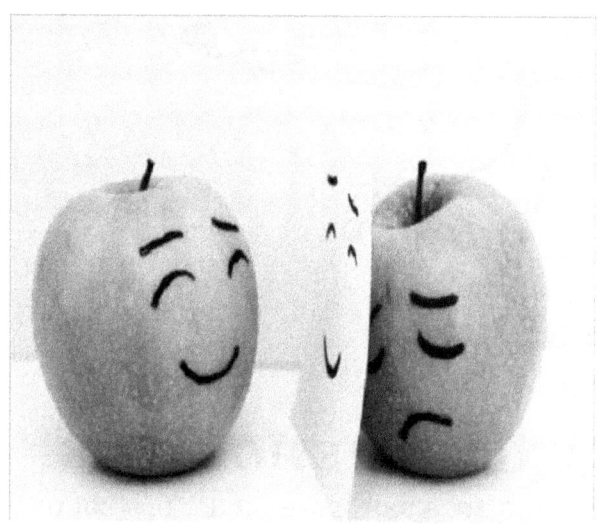

DEALING WITH HOLIDAY DEPRESSION

For those who have lost a spouse or significant other, there are several other ways to get rid of the holiday blues including:

Begin a new tradition. Plan a family outing or vacation instead of spending the holidays at home.

Don't succumb to holiday pressures. Feel free to leave an event if you aren't comfortable, and be willing to tell others. "I'm not up for this right now."

Volunteer. Work at a soup kitchen, organize a gift drive, or simply help the neighbor dig the snow out of their driveway.

Get back to nature. Going for a walk in the park or the woods helps many people who are feeling overwhelmed to feel better.

Chapter 5

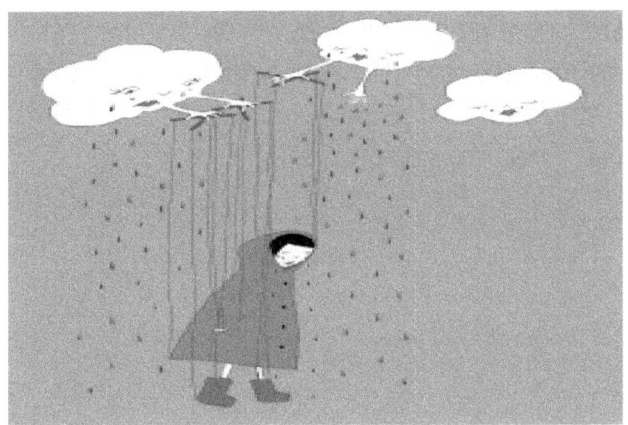

MOST COMMON CAUSES OF HOLIDAY DEPRESSION

When the colder weather sets in and the holidays roll around, many people experience a change in mood that can sometimes escalate to depression. This type of holiday depression, while common, can be caused by many different factors in an individual's life. For some it may be one single issue causing the depression, but for others, it can be a combination of many things that they are struggling with. Now you'll learn the possible causes of holiday depression so you will know what signs to look for if you think you may be suffering from this condition.

What is Holiday Depression?

The winter season and the holidays are one time of the year when many people become especially vulnerable to depression. This is a condition that may affect a person only for the duration of the season, or it may simply be a trigger for depression that could extend beyond the winter or the holidays. In addition to or separate from this condition, some people suffer from **Seasonal Affective Disorder** (SAD), which is a seasonal type of depression connected to changes in the weather. With both types of these conditions, symptoms like loss of energy, sluggishness, increased appetite, irritability and unhappiness are common symptoms.

Chapter 6

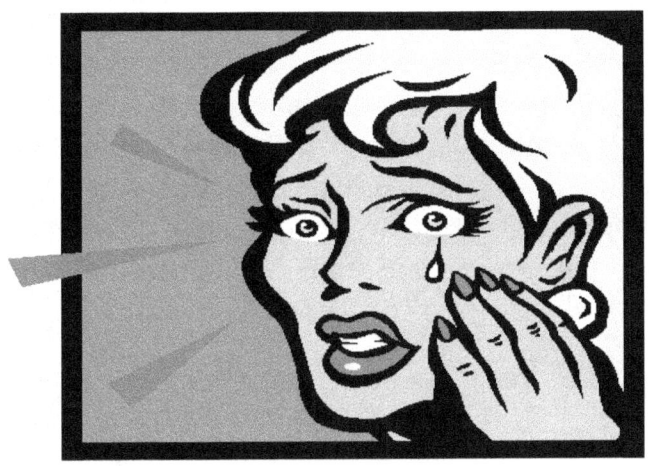

CHALLENGES OF HOLIDAY DEPRESSION

One of the challenges with holiday depression, and seasonal affective disorder is that there are so many different possible causes. Among the many potential triggers for this condition are:

Stress: The holidays, while a time for celebration, can be a huge source of stress for many people. One factor can be shopping for gifts, which take up time, involve dealing with crowds and traffic, and the pressure of deciding what to get for your loved ones. Additionally, many people may experience anxiety about how much money they are spending. Stress can also stem from organizing family get-togethers, making sure holiday cards are sent out on time, and dozens of other things that make holiday schedules packed to the brim.

Fatigue: Along with packed holiday schedules comes exhaustion, which many people have to deal with during this season. Fatigue is a common contributing factor to holiday depression since it leads to a lack of exercise, not wanting to leave the house, and may even lead to a weakened immune system.

Family-Related Issues: Some people rarely see their families outside of the holidays, which may make this particular season a little more difficult to deal with than others. Spending time with parents, siblings, and other relatives can cause tension in some families, and the anxiety of these get-togethers can also be a trigger for depression.

Loneliness: While some are experiencing family issues, other people have trouble during the holidays for the opposite reason. Not being able to spend time with loved ones due to financial constraints, distance, or other reasons can cause severe loneliness during the holidays. Also, those who have family members or friends who have passed away may miss them even more during special times like the holidays.

Unrealistic Expectations: Some people get overly excited about the holidays, but when the reality of the events set in, they may find themselves disappointed with the actual outcome. Whether it's holiday parties not being as much fun as hoped for, loved ones not getting as excited about their gifts as you'd hoped, or other bad experiences, the sadness of a holiday season that doesn't match up with an individual's idea of what a picture-perfect holiday season should be like.

Reduced Sunlight: The lack of sunlight during the winter months can be one of the triggers for seasonal affective disorder. In addition to affective chemical balances within the body, longer periods of darkness can also make a person less likely to want to go outside, exercise, or spend time with others. Because of this symptom, special forms of light therapy have been developed to allow those with SAD to get the light exposure that they need.

If you think that you may be suffering holiday depression, or seasonal affective disorder, see a doctor or a therapist right away. There are several ways of dealing with or treating these conditions that can help you get through the winter and the holidays.

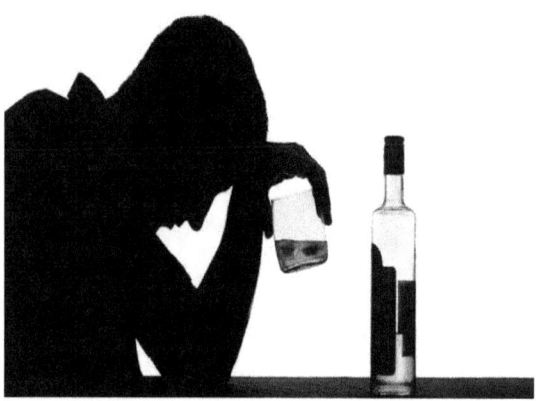

Chapter 7

HOW TO OVERCOME HOLIDAY DEPRESSION AND ADDICTION

The holidays may look like a Norman Rockwell painting for many, but the stress and strain of the season makes some people feel anything but cheery and bright. According to the Mental health American, as many as 12 percent of Americans, a large percentage of them women, experience holiday depression and suffer from "seasonal affective disorder" (SAD).

According to the MHA, depression during holidays can be caused by "stress, fatigue, unrealistic expectations, over-commercialization, financial constraints, or the inability to be with one's family and friends". Here are some helpful tips on how to prevent the holiday blues from creeping in, and how to overcome existing holiday depression and addiction.

Don't Overextend Yourself

The mistake many Americans make during the holidays is overextending them-selves. They commit to more parties than they can actually attend, they purchase more gifts than they can afford, and they are not realistic about what they can or cannot accomplish during the holiday season. Keep your expectations for the season manageable by setting realistic goals for yourself, organizing your time, and making lists that prioritize important activities.

If you are feeling overwhelmed during the holiday season, chances are you are too stress, and you have forgotten that the holidays are supposed to be fun. If you find yourself having one of these stressful moments, take some time to yourself. Don't worry about rushing around, finishing your shopping, planning the menu or finishing the cooking - just stop, breathe, and take a moment to be calm. If you do not take the time to enjoy your family, friends and the beautiful season, then what is the point?

On the other hand, we all know that the holidays become more and more commercialized as the years go by, and a lot of the things people feel obligated to do during the holiday season can easily turn into a source of stress.

Therapist understands why the holidays and depression are often synonymous. "Holidays may remind you that you are away from those you truly love, or that you are not making as much money as you'd like, or that you're not romantically linked to someone to share in the joy and the misery of the season". It is also important to realize that many people are in the same boat as you; everyone has limitations as to how much they can spend and how many parties they can attend. Try only cooking and purchasing gifts for close family and friends, only attend parties that you are sincerely excited and happy to attend – don't make yourself miserable by putting yourself in debt, and surrounding yourself with people that you do not truly want to spend the holidays with.

Acknowledge Your Feelings

The holidays, though fun and exciting, can also bring a great deal of stress. The feeling that you are not alone in this, and that many others across the country are feeling the same stress can be very helpful in overcoming holiday depression.

If you're not able to spend as much money as you would like on gifts for your loved ones, or if you have more on your plate than you can handle, that would exhaust and stress anyone out. It's important that you know it's ok to feel the way you're feeling and also, that it's normal to feel those things around this time of year". Professional therapist say.

There are many Americans who cannot be home for the holidays because they are deployed outside of the United States, they cannot get away from work, or they simply cannot afford to make it home to their families for the various holidays. Acknowledging feelings of longing and loneliness and; knowing that it is acceptable to feel this way during the holidays is helpful for those grappling with holiday depression associated with being away from loved ones.

The Mental Health Association (MHA) asks those struggling with these feelings to remember that the holiday season does not banish reasons for feeling sad or lonely, and that there is room for these feelings to be present, even if certain individuals choose not to express them.

Other helpful suggestions include spending time with supportive and caring people, reaching out and making new friends, or contacting someone you have not heard from in a while. We've have all heard the saying that laughter is the best medicine, old friends and new friends alike can be very helpful in avoiding or curing depression during the holidays.

Oftentimes, talking to people who are going through similar situations, or who are experiencing similar feelings can prove to be very helpful in overcoming your own sadness during this otherwise happy time of year. Bonding over shared feelings of holiday depression, or perhaps opening up to a new friend capable of understanding your situation can also be very beneficial to your well being during this emotionally exhaustive time of year.

Don't Make It Worse

If you are already suffering from holiday depression, you may be more apt to overindulge in some of the more unhealthy aspects of the holiday season, such as rich fatty food, large amounts of alcohol, or spending beyond your means in order to feel better about your current situation.

The MHA refers to acting out in these ways as "stress responses". Many people find comfort in food, having a few drinks, or in shopping, however, engaging in these activities to excess during the holiday season in order to de-stress will only make the situation worse. It is important that you deal with your holiday depression in a healthy way because if you don't it can result in more depression. Many people experience what is commonly referred to as "post holiday let down" after New Year's, meaning that the disappointments during the preceding months are compounded by the excess fatigue and stress they feel due to increased debt, extra weight, or a new-found dependency on alcohol.

Nothing makes holiday depression worse than dwelling on it. Rather than fixating on things you cannot change, or feeling sorry for yourself during the holiday season, try doing something that makes you feel productive, and better about your-self. "Going jogging, taking your dog to the park, making holiday crafts with your kids-these are instant, costless, productive and healthy ways to get your mind off things, and get you feeling good again."

Also, therapist suggest volunteering at a shelter, taking part in charitable organizations, or doing something as simple as helping a friend in need. It is easy to get lost in the hustle and bustle of the season, and all of us can say that at one time or another, we have been guilty of forgetting the true meaning of the season, and instead of fixating on what can only be described as luxuries by those in need. Nothing will put such trivial matters in perspective like helping those who are less fortunate. No matter how little you think you have, there are always those who have less, and volunteering somewhere will drive that point home. It is also important to understand that the intention of volunteering is not to make you feel guilty about what you have; instead, it should make you feel grateful.

Feelings of depression during holidays can seem overwhelming. During this busy time of year, spend time with those you love, and remember not to sweat the small stuff. You can't buy happiness or good health, so focus on fixing the things you can fix, and forget about things that are beyond your control.

Set aside differences. Try to accept family members and friends as they are, even if they don't live up to all of your expectations. Set aside grievances until a more appropriate time for discussion. And be understanding if others get upset or distressed when something goes wrong. Chances are they're feeling the effects of holiday stress and depression too.

Take a breather. Make some time for yourself. Spending just 15 minutes alone, without distractions, may refresh you enough to handle everything you need to do. Find something that reduces stress by clearing your mind, slowing your breathing, and restoring inner calm. Some options may include:

Taking a walk at night and stargazing.

Listening to soothing music.

Getting a massage.

Reading a book.

Plan ahead. Set aside specific days for shopping, baking, visiting friends, and other activities. Plan your menus and then make your shopping list. That'll help prevent last-minute scrambling to buy forgotten ingredients. And make sure to line up help for party prep and cleanup.

Seek professional help if you need it. Despite your best efforts, you may find yourself feeling persistently sad or anxious, plagued by physical complaints, unable to sleep, irritable and hopeless, and unable to face routine chores. If these feelings last for a while, talk to your doctor, or a mental health professional.

Take control of the holidays. Don't let the holidays become something you dread. Instead, take steps to prevent the stress and depression that can descend during the holidays. Learn to recognize your holiday triggers, such as financial pressures, or personal demands, so you can combat them before they lead to a meltdown. With a little planning and some positive thinking, you can find peace and joy during the holidays.

Conclusion

Thank you again for choosing this book!

I hope this book was able to help you to overcome depression and addictions and enjoy the holidays.

Don't get hung up on what the holidays are supposed to be like, and how you're supposed to feel. If you're comparing your holidays to some abstract greeting card ideal, they'll always come up short. So don't worry about holiday spirit and take the holidays as they come.

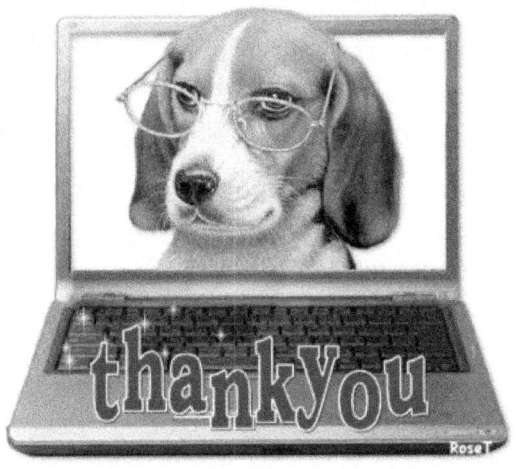

Finally, if you enjoyed this book, would you be kind enough to leave a review for this book on Amazon? It'd be greatly appreciated!

Thank you and good luck!

Preview Of 'THE DEPRESSION CURE: How to Overcome Depression and Become Depression Free'

Chapter 1: MOOD DISORDER

Tackling depression head-on the right way

Recovery begins when we overcome depression and become totally depression free. Treatment for depression starts when one recognizes the symptoms and began to seek help. To find a Depression cure it requires patience from both the individual and the physician. Depression is not like normal sadness and happiness if you are experiencing feelings of despair, or hopelessness. Most people do not realize they are depressed and let this illness go unnoticed. However, it may be because they don't know the warning signs or the triggers of their depression. When you're feeling lonely, and not able to socialize, you should try taking a walk or sharing your company with someone you trust. Good conversation can be refreshing and uplifting once again. Also, when you feel your thoughts and feelings, and your sense of well being have disappeared, try taking make you happy. Finding a cure for depression, unlike relief from stress does not time out for yourself and go on a vacation, or find something that you know will happen naturally.

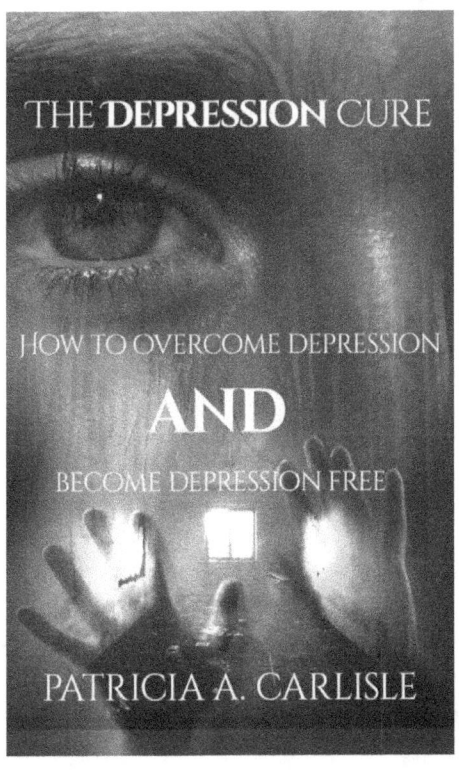

To check out the rest of (THE DEPRESSION CURE: How to Overcome Depression and Become Depression Free) go to amazon.com

Check Out My Other Books

Below you'll find some of my other popular books that are popular on Amazon and Kindle as well. Alternatively, you can visit my author page on Amazon to see other work done by me. (https://amazon.com/author/patriciacarlisle)

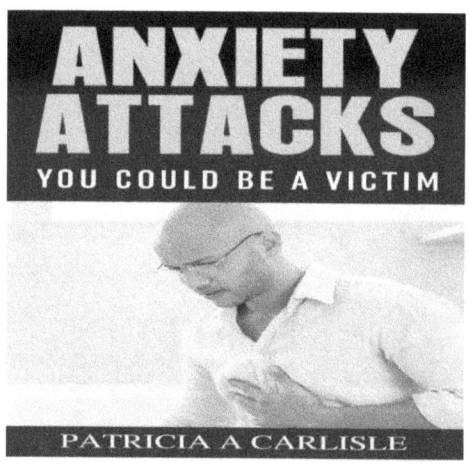

ANXIETY ATTACKS: YOU COULD BE A VICTIM.

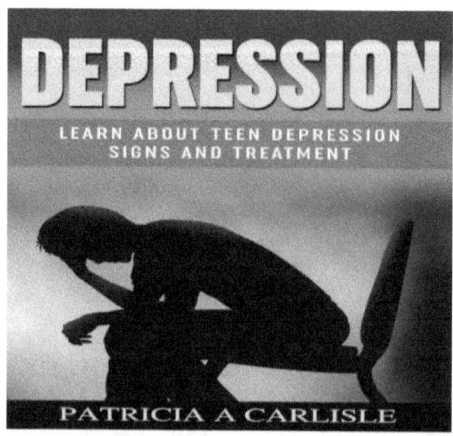

DEPRESSION: Learn About Teen Depression Signs and Treatment.

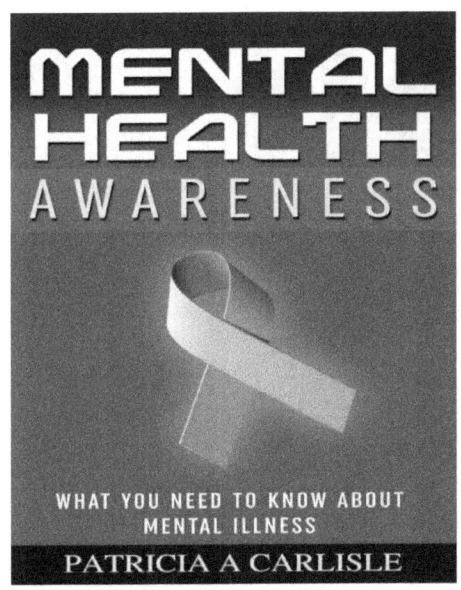

MENTAL HEALTH AWARENESS: What You Need To Know About Mental Illness.

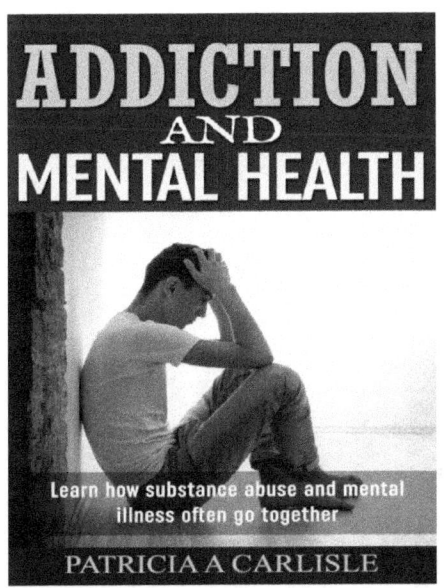

ADDICTION AND MENTAL HEALTH: Learn How Substance Abuse and Mental Illness Often Go Together.

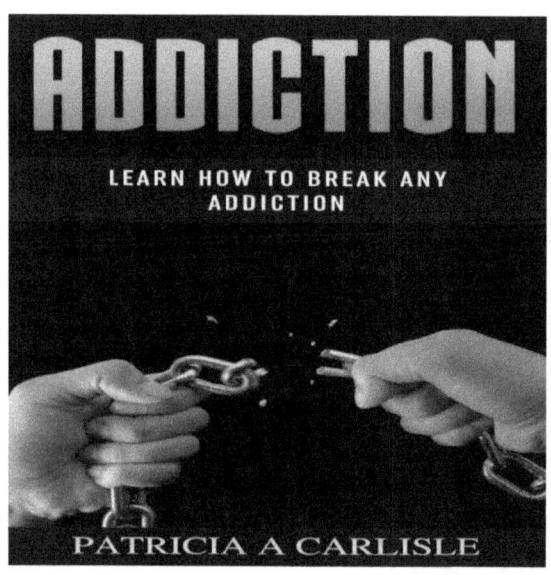

ADDICTION: Learn How To Break Any Addiction.

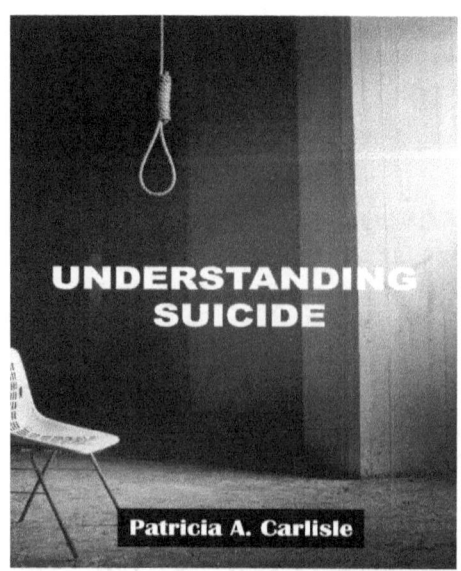

UNDERSTANDING SUICIDE.

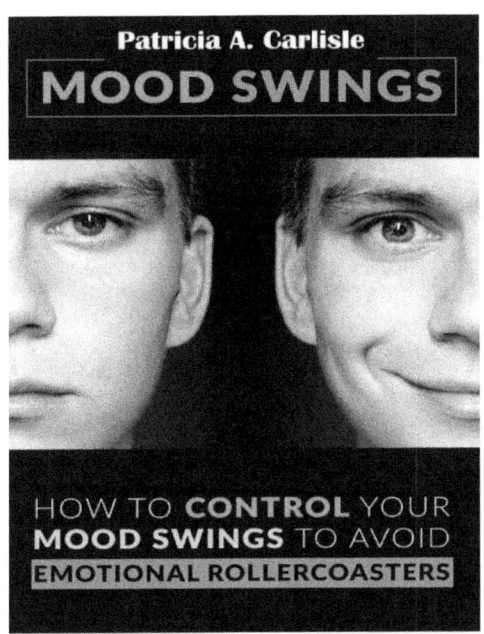

MOOD SWINGS: How to Control Your Mood Swings to Avoid Emotional Rollercoaster's.

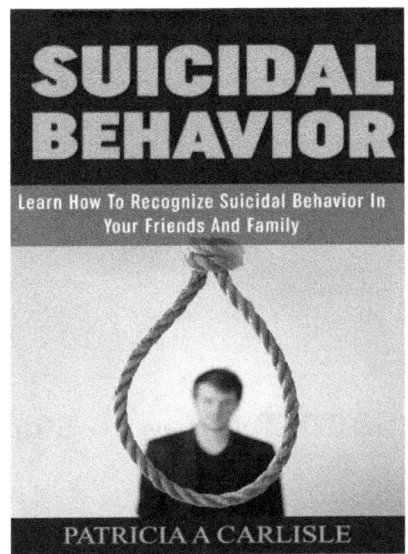

SUICIDAL BEHAVIOR: Learn How To Recognize Suicidal Behavior In Your Friends and Family.

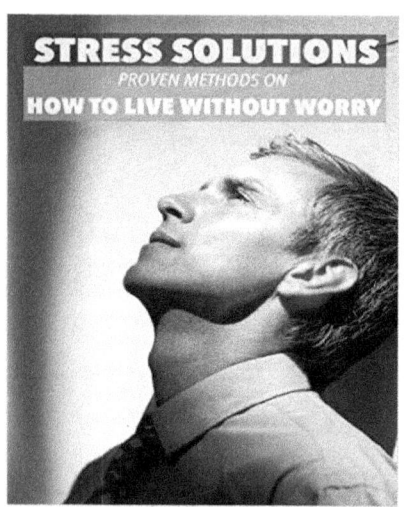

STRESS SOLUTIONS: Proven Methods On How To Live Without Worry.

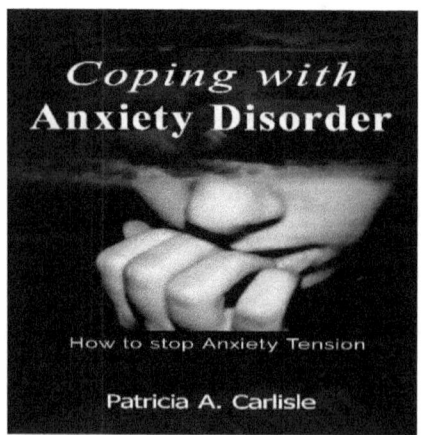

COPING WITH ANXIETY DISORDER: How to Stop Anxiety Tension.

You can simply search for these titles on the Amazon website to find them.

BONUS: SUBSCRIBE TO THE FREE BOOK

Beginners Guide to Yoga & Meditation

"Stressed out? Do You Feel Like The World Is Crashing Down Around You? Want To Take A Vacation That Will Relax Your Mind, Body And Spirit? Well this Easy To Read Step By Step

E-Book Makes It All Possible!"

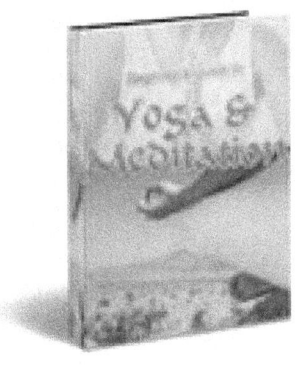

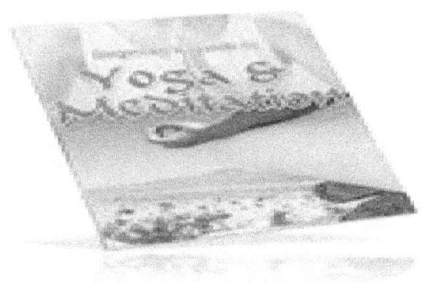

Instructions on how to join our mailing list, and receive a free copy of "Yoga and Meditation" can be found in any of my Kindle eBooks.

NOTES

NOTES

NOTES

NOTES

NOTES